MACRO COOKBOOK FOR BEGINNERS

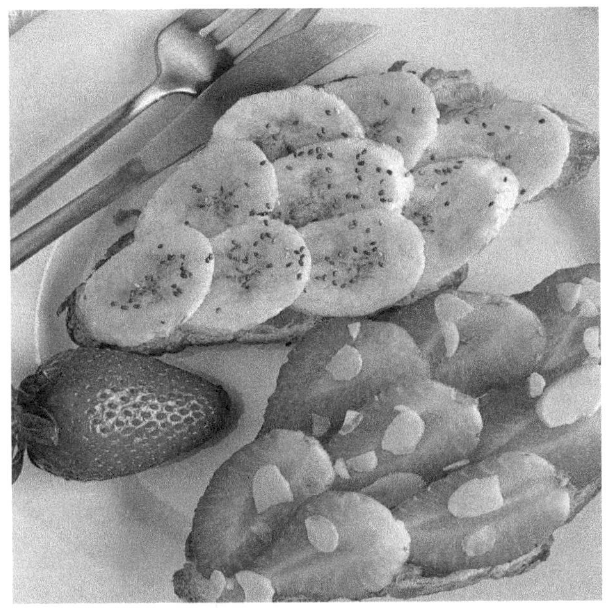

A Comprehensive Guide with Over 320 Recipes for Body Metabolism

Francisco pace

Table of Content

Introduction

Once upon a time, in a bustling city nestled between towering skyscrapers and bustling streets, there lived a young aspiring chef named Emma. Emma had always been fascinated by the art of cooking, but she found herself particularly drawn to the world of macro cooking - the delicate balance of nutrients and flavors that could transform ordinary ingredients into extraordinary meals.

Growing up, Emma had watched her grandmother whip up delicious meals from scratch, carefully measuring each ingredient and paying close attention to the nutritional value of every dish. Inspired by her grandmother's culinary prowess, Emma set out on a quest to master the art of macro cooking.

Armed with her trusty apron and a collection of recipes passed down through generations, Emma embarked on her journey to become a macro cooking master. She spent hours poring over cookbooks and scouring the internet for tips and tricks to elevate her skills in the kitchen.

As Emma experimented with different ingredients and techniques, she quickly learned that macro cooking was more than just following recipes - it was a culinary adventure that required creativity, precision, and a keen understanding of nutrition. With each dish she created, Emma honed her skills and expanded her repertoire, delighting friends and family with her flavorful creations.

But Emma knew that there was still so much to learn. Determined to take her macro cooking to the next level, she sought out the wisdom of seasoned chefs and nutrition experts, eager to soak up their knowledge and expertise.

Through countless hours of practice and perseverance, Emma began to develop her own unique style of macro cooking - a harmonious blend of fresh ingredients, bold flavors, and balanced nutrients. Her dishes were not only delicious but also nourishing, fueling both body and soul with every bite.

As word of Emma's culinary talents spread, she realized that she had a gift to share with the world. And so, she set out to create her very own macro cookbook for beginners - a comprehensive guide to mastering the art of macro cooking, filled with easy-to-follow recipes, helpful tips, and insightful advice.

With each page of her cookbook, Emma sought to empower aspiring chefs to embrace the world of macro cooking and unlock their full culinary potential. From hearty breakfasts to satisfying dinners, Emma's recipes were designed to cater to every palate and dietary preference, ensuring that everyone could enjoy the benefits of delicious and nutritious meals. But Emma's journey was far from over. As she continued to explore the endless possibilities of macro cooking, she discovered new ingredients, techniques, and flavors that inspired her to push the boundaries of her creativity even further.

And so, armed with her trusty cookbook and an insatiable appetite for culinary adventure, Emma embarked on her next chapter - spreading the joy of macro cooking far and wide, one delicious dish at a time. For Emma knew that with passion, perseverance, and a dash of creativity, anyone could become a master of macro cooking.

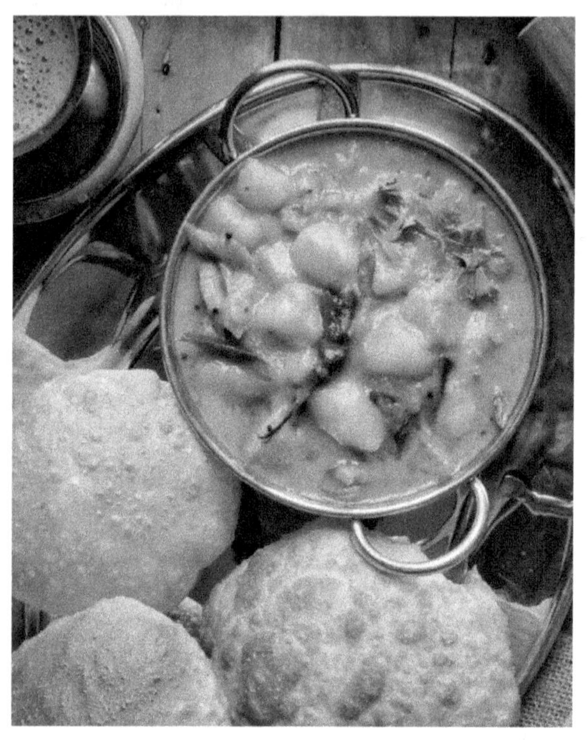

Mashed Potatoes Soup

Chapter One

macronutrients

Macronutrients are essential nutrients required by the body in relatively large amounts to maintain proper function, growth, and health. There are three primary macronutrients:

1.	**Carbohydrate**: The body uses carbs as its main energy source. Cells use glucose, which is produced when they are broken down, as fuel. Carbohydrates also play a role in providing dietary fiber, which aids in digestion and helps maintain healthy bowel function. Carbs are commonly found in grains, fruits, vegetables, and legumes. Sugars, starches, and fiber are the three primary categories of carbohydrates.
There are two other types of sugars: simple sugars, which are present in fruits, honey, and refined sugars, and complex sugars, which are present in grains and starchy vegetables.

Complex carbohydrates, or starches, are present in foods like grains, legumes, and starchy vegetables like corn and potatoes.

2. **Proteins**: Proteins are essential for building and repairing tissues, as well as for the production of enzymes, hormones, and other important molecules in the body. Proteins are made up of amino acids, some of which are produced by the body (non-essential amino acids), while others must be obtained from the diet (essential amino acids).
Meat, poultry, fish, eggs, dairy products, legumes, nuts, and seeds are all excellent sources of protein. Proteins are made up of chains of amino acids, which are essential for numerous bodily functions.

There are 20 amino acids, nine of which are essential, meaning the body cannot produce them and must obtain them from the diet.

Animal sources of protein, such as meat, poultry, fish, eggs, and dairy products, typically provide all essential amino acids in adequate amounts. These are regarded as protein wholly.

2.   **Fats**: Fats are a concentrated source of energy and are essential for various bodily functions, including providing insulation, cushioning organs, and facilitating the absorption of fat-soluble vitamins (such as

vitamins A, D, E, and K). Fats are also important for cell membrane structure and hormone production.There are several kinds of fats: trans fats, monounsaturated and polyunsaturated unsaturated fats, and saturated fats. Healthy sources of fats include avocados, nuts, seeds, olive oil, fatty fish, and coconut oil.

These macronutrients are required in varying amounts depending on factors such as age, sex, weight, activity level, and overall health status. For optimum health and wellbeing, a diet rich in a variety of foods high in carbs, proteins, and fats must be balanced.

 Fats are composed of fatty acids, which can be classified as saturated, unsaturated (monounsaturated and polyunsaturated), and trans fats.
- Saturated fats are solid at room temperature and are primarily found in animal products such as meat, dairy, and certain plant oils like coconut and palm oil. High consumption of saturated fats has been linked to elevated cholesterol and an increased risk of heart disease.

Unsaturated fats, including monounsaturated and polyunsaturated fats, are liquid at room temperature and are considered healthier options. They are found in foods like olive oil, avocado, nuts, seeds, and fatty fish.

Trans fats are artificial fats created through a process called hydrogenation and are commonly found in processed and fried foods. They are known to increase the risk of heart disease and should be avoided as much as possible.

Balancing the intake of these macronutrients is essential for maintaining optimal health and preventing chronic diseases It is noteworthy that the dietary requirements of individuals may differ, and seeking advice from a healthcare practitioner or qualified dietitian can offer tailored counsel.

Importance of Macro nutrients

Macronutrients are essential components of the human diet, providing the body with energy and supporting various physiological functions. These nutrients include carbohydrates, proteins, and fats, each playing a crucial role in maintaining overall health and well-being.

Carbohydrates:
Carbohydrates are the body's primary source of energy, providing fuel for various activities ranging from basic bodily functions to intense physical exercise. They are composed of carbon, hydrogen, and oxygen atoms and are

categorized into simple and complex carbohydrates.

Energy Production: Carbohydrates are broken down into glucose, which is readily utilized by cells for energy production through processes like glycolysis and the citric acid cycle.
Brain Function: Glucose is the preferred fuel for the brain, supporting cognitive function, concentration, and mental clarity.

Muscle Fuel: During exercise, carbohydrates stored as glycogen in muscles provide energy for prolonged physical activity.

Dietary Sources: Common sources include grains, fruits, vegetables, legumes, and dairy products.

Carbohydrates encompass a broad range of compounds, including sugars, starches, and fiber. While often vilified in popular diets, carbohydrates are essential for optimal health when consumed in appropriate quantities and from nutritious sources.

Fiber: A significant component of carbohydrates, fiber plays a crucial role in digestive health, promoting regular bowel movements, preventing constipation, and reducing the risk of colon cancer. Additionally, soluble fiber helps lower cholesterol levels and stabilize blood sugar levels, contributing to heart health and diabetes management.

Glycemic Index: Carbohydrate-containing foods vary in their glycemic index (GI), a measure of how quickly they raise blood sugar levels. Choosing low-GI carbohydrates can help regulate blood sugar levels, improve satiety, and reduce the risk of insulin resistance and type 2 diabetes.

Fuel for Endurance Exercise: For athletes and individuals engaged in prolonged or intense physical activity, carbohydrates are essential for maintaining energy levels and enhancing performance. Carbohydrate-loading strategies before endurance events can maximize glycogen stores in muscles and liver, delaying fatigue and improving endurance capacity.

 Proteins:
Proteins are fundamental to the structure and function of cells, tissues, and organs in the body. They are composed of amino acids, which are linked together in various sequences to form specific proteins.

Tissue Building: Proteins serve as the building blocks for muscles, bones, skin, hair, and nails, playing a crucial role in tissue repair and growth.
Enzyme Function: Many enzymes, which facilitate biochemical reactions in the body, are composed of proteins.
Immune Support: Antibodies, essential components of the immune system, are proteins that help defend the body against infections and diseases.
Hormone Regulation: Certain hormones, such as insulin and growth hormone, are proteins that regulate various physiological processes.

Dietary Sources: Complete protein sources include meat, poultry, fish, eggs, dairy, and soy products, while incomplete sources include grains, legumes, nuts, and seeds.

Fats:
Fats, also known as lipids, are highly concentrated sources of energy and play critical roles in cell structure, hormone production, and nutrient absorption. They are composed of carbon, hydrogen, and oxygen atoms and are categorized into saturated, unsaturated, and trans fats.

Energy Storage: Fats provide a dense source of energy, with each gram containing more than twice the calories of carbohydrates or proteins. They serve as a long-term energy reserve, stored in adipose tissue throughout the body.

Cellular Structure: Phospholipids, a type of lipid, are essential components of cell membranes, maintaining their integrity and facilitating communication between cells.

Hormone Production: Cholesterol, a type of lipid, serves as a precursor for the synthesis of steroid hormones, including cortisol, estrogen, and testosterone.

Vitamin Absorption: Certain vitamins, such as A, D, E, and K, are fat-soluble, meaning they require fat for absorption and transportation within the body.

Dietary Sources: Healthy sources of fats include avocados, nuts, seeds, olive oil, fatty fish, and coconut oil, while unhealthy sources include fried foods, processed snacks, and high-fat dairy products.
Fats are a diverse group of molecules that serve as a concentrated source of energy and contribute to numerous physiological functions, despite their reputation as a dietary villain in some circles.

Omega-3 Fatty Acids: Found primarily in fatty fish, flaxseeds, and walnuts, omega-3 fatty acids are essential for heart health, brain function, and inflammation regulation. Adequate intake of these polyunsaturated fats has been associated with a reduced risk of cardiovascular disease, cognitive decline, and inflammatory conditions.

Cell Signaling: Lipids play crucial roles in cell signaling and communication, modulating processes such as inflammation, immune response, and gene expression. Certain lipid molecules, such as prostaglandins and leukotrienes, regulate inflammation and immune function, influencing the body's response to injury and infection.

Cholesterol Regulation: While often demonized for its role in cardiovascular disease, cholesterol is a vital lipid molecule involved in cell membrane integrity, hormone production, and bile acid synthesis. Maintaining a balance between "good" (HDL) and "bad" (LDL) cholesterol levels is essential for heart health and overall well-being.

Balanced Macronutrient Intake:

Achieving a balanced intake of macronutrients is essential for overall health and well-being. While the specific proportions may vary based on individual factors such as age, gender, activity level, and metabolic rate, a general guideline is to consume a diet consisting of approximately:

45-65% Carbohydrates: Emphasizing complex carbohydrates such as whole grains, fruits, and vegetables while limiting refined sugars and processed foods.

10-35% Proteins: Including a variety of lean protein sources such as poultry, fish, legumes, and plant-based proteins to support tissue repair and growth.

20-35% Fats: Prioritizing unsaturated fats from sources like nuts, seeds, and olive oil while minimizing saturated and trans fats from processed and fried foods.

macronutrients are vital components of the human diet, providing energy and supporting various physiological functions essential for health and well-being. Carbohydrates serve as the body's primary energy source, proteins are crucial for tissue repair and growth, and fats play diverse roles in cellular structure, hormone production, and nutrient absorption. Achieving a balanced intake of macronutrients is key to optimizing health and preventing diet-related diseases, emphasizing whole foods and minimizing processed and refined products. By understanding the importance of macronutrients and making informed dietary choices, individuals can enhance their overall quality of life and promote longevity.

Nutrient Timing and Distribution:

In addition to considering the types and quantities of macronutrients consumed, the timing and distribution of nutrient intake throughout the day can impact metabolic processes, energy levels, and overall health outcomes.

Meal Frequency: While traditional dietary guidelines often recommend three square meals per day, some individuals may benefit from more frequent, smaller meals or snacks to maintain energy levels, stabilize blood sugar, and support metabolism.

Pre- and Post-Exercise Nutrition: Consuming a balanced meal or snack containing carbohydrates and protein before and after exercise can optimize performance, enhance recovery, and promote muscle protein synthesis. Carbohydrates provide immediate energy, while protein supports muscle repair and growth.

Macronutrient Ratios

 While general guidelines exist for macronutrient distribution, individual needs may vary based on factors such as age, gender, body composition, activity level, and metabolic rate. Experimenting with different macronutrient ratios can help individuals identify the optimal balance for their unique goals and preferences.

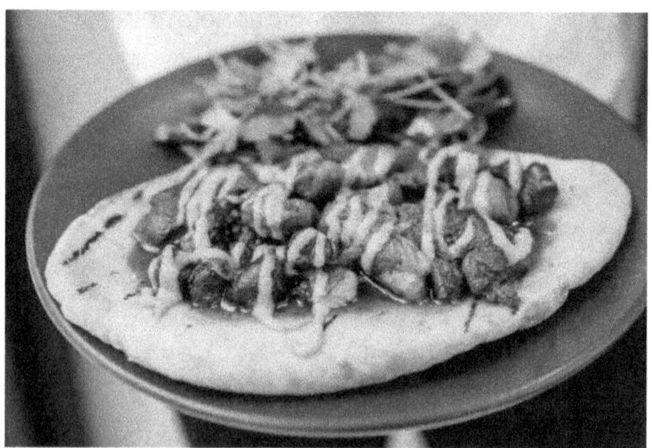

Chapter Two

Determining your Daily Calorie need

Determining your daily calorie intake involves understanding your Basal Metabolic Rate (BMR), which is the amount of energy your body needs to maintain basic functions at rest, and factoring in your activity level and any goals you have, such as weight loss or maintenance.

1. **Basal Metabolic Rate (BMR)**: This is the energy your body needs to function at rest. Factors including height, weight, gender, and age have an impact on it. One commonly used formula to estimate BMR is the Harris-Benedict Equation, which takes into account these factors. Your BMR represents the calories your body burns at rest to maintain vital functions like breathing, circulating blood, and regulating body temperature. Various formulas can estimate BMR, such as the Mifflin-St Jeor equation or the Katch-McArdle formula, which consider factors like age, gender,

weight, and height. Understanding your BMR provides a baseline for determining your calorie needs.

2. **Activity Level**: Once you have your BMR, you need to factor in your activity level using the Total Daily Energy Expenditure (TDEE) formula. This includes physical activity and exercise. There are different activity level categories, from sedentary (little to no exercise) to very active (intense exercise multiple times a week). Identifying your activity level is crucial for accurately calculating your Total Daily Energy Expenditure (TDEE), which encompasses both your BMR and the calories burned through physical activity. Sedentary individuals have little to no exercise, while those who are very active engage in intense physical activity regularly. Your activity level helps adjust your calorie intake based on how much energy you expend throughout the day.

3. **Goals**: Depending on your goals, you adjust your calorie intake. For weight maintenance, your intake matches your TDEE. For weight loss, you create a calorie deficit by consuming fewer calories than your TDEE, typically 500 to 1000 calories less per day for a steady weight loss of 1 to

2 pounds per week. For weight gain, you consume more calories than your TDEE. Dietary changes and increased physical exercise can be combined to accomplish this shortfall. Conversely, for weight gain, you need to consume more calories than your TDEE, focusing on nutrient-rich foods to support muscle growth and overall health.

4. **Monitoring and Adjusting**: Regularly monitoring your progress is essential to ensure you're on track with your goals. This involves tracking your calorie intake, physical activity, and weight changes over time. If you're not seeing the desired results, adjustments may be needed, such as tweaking your calorie intake or reassessing your activity level. It's a dynamic process that requires flexibility and willingness to adapt as needed.

5. **Quality of Calories**: While the quantity of calories is important for weight management, so is the quality. Aim for a balanced diet with nutrient-dense foods to ensure you're meeting your body's nutritional needs.

Aim to prioritize nutrient-dense foods that provide essential vitamins, minerals, and macronutrients while minimizing processed foods high in added sugars and unhealthy fats. Focusing on whole foods, such as fruits, vegetables, lean proteins, whole grains, and healthy fats, supports optimal nutrition and satiety.

6.   **Consistency**: Consistency is the cornerstone of successful calorie management. Establishing consistent eating patterns, exercise routines, and lifestyle habits helps regulate appetite, energy levels, and metabolic function. Strive for balance, moderation, and sustainability in your approach to calorie intake, making gradual changes that you can maintain long-term.

By considering these factors and incorporating them into your daily routine, you can effectively determine and manage your calorie intake to support your health and fitness goals.

Adjusting macros for specific Goals : weight Loss, Muscle gain, maintenance

Adjusting macros for specific goals like weight loss, muscle gain, and maintenance involves tailoring your macronutrient intake to support those objectives. Here's a detailed explanation for each:

Weight Loss:
1. Caloric Deficit: To lose weight, you need to consume fewer calories than you expend. Adjust your macros to support this deficit.

2. Protein: Increase protein intake to preserve lean muscle mass while losing fat. Aim for 0.7-1 gram of protein per pound of body weight.

3. Carbohydrates: Reduce carbohydrate intake, especially refined carbs and sugars, to control blood sugar levels and promote fat loss.

4. Fats: Include healthy fats like avocados, nuts, and olive oil to support satiety and overall health, but moderate intake to control calorie consumption.

 Muscle Gain:
1. Caloric Surplus: Consume more calories than you burn to support muscle growth. Adjust macros to ensure sufficient energy for workouts and recovery.

2. Protein: Increase protein intake to support muscle repair and growth.Per pound of body weight, aim for a protein intake of 1–1.5 grams.

3. Carbohydrates: Increase carbohydrate intake to fuel workouts and replenish glycogen stores. Choose complex carbohydrates such as fruits, vegetables, and whole grains.

4. Fats: Include healthy fats to support hormone production and overall health, but prioritize carbohydrates and protein for energy and muscle growth.

Maintenance:

1. Caloric Balance: Consume the same amount of calories as you expend to maintain current weight. Adjust macros to maintain energy levels and overall health.

2. Protein: Maintain protein intake at a moderate level to support muscle maintenance and overall health. Aim for 0.6-0.8 grams of protein per pound of body weight.

3. Carbohydrates: Balance carbohydrate intake to meet energy needs without excess. Focus on whole food sources to support overall health and satiety.

4. Fats: Continue including healthy fats in moderation to support nutrient absorption

and hormone regulation without exceeding caloric needs.

 individual needs may vary based on factors like activity level, metabolism, and body composition. It's essential to monitor progress and adjust macros accordingly for optimal results. Consulting with a registered dietitian or nutritionist can provide personalized guidance based on your specific goals and requirements.

Setting macro nutrients ratio for proteins, carbohydrates and fat and oil.

Setting the macronutrient ratio for proteins, carbohydrates, and fats is essential for achieving specific dietary goals, whether it's weight loss, muscle gain, or general health maintenance. The optimal ratio varies based on individual factors such as age, gender, activity level, metabolic rate, and specific health goals. However, there are some general guidelines and principles to consider when determining the ideal macronutrient ratio.

1. Proteins: Building and mending tissues, generating hormones and enzymes, and bolstering immune system function all depend on proteins. The recommended

dietary allowance (RDA) for protein intake is 0.8 grams per kilogram of body weight per day for sedentary individuals. However, athletes, those looking to build muscle, or individuals on a weight loss journey may require higher protein intake.

 - For sedentary individuals: 10-15% of total daily calories.
 - For athletes or those engaging in intense physical activity: 15-25% of total daily calories.
 - For individuals on a high-protein diet for weight loss: 25-35% of total daily calories. Lean meats, poultry, fish, eggs, dairy products, legumes, nuts, and seeds are among the foods that are rich in protein. It's essential to choose a variety of protein sources to ensure adequate intake of essential amino acids.

2. Carbohydrates:
   Carbohydrates are the body's primary source of energy, especially for high-intensity exercise and brain function. However, not all carbohydrates are created equal. Complex carbohydrates, such as whole grains, fruits, vegetables, and legumes, provide fiber, vitamins, and minerals, while simple carbohydrates, like sugar and refined grains, offer little nutritional value.

- For general health and weight maintenance: 45-65% of total daily calories.
- For endurance athletes or those engaging in prolonged exercise: 55-65% of total daily calories.
- For individuals on a low-carb or ketogenic diet: 5-10% of total daily calories.

Emphasizing whole, unprocessed carbohydrates over refined and sugary foods is crucial for maintaining stable blood sugar levels, sustained energy, and overall health.

3. Fats and Oils:
Fats play various roles in the body, including providing energy, supporting cell growth, protecting organs, and aiding in the absorption of fat-soluble vitamins (A, D, E, and K). However, not all fats are created equal. Unsaturated fats, found in foods like avocados, nuts, seeds, and olive oil, are considered heart-healthy and should be prioritized over saturated and trans fats.

- For general health and weight maintenance: 20-35% of total daily calories.
- For individuals on a high-fat or ketogenic diet: 60-75% of total daily calories.

It's essential to focus on incorporating unsaturated fats, including

monounsaturated and polyunsaturated fats, into the diet while minimizing intake of saturated and trans fats, commonly found in processed and fried foods.

In determining the optimal macronutrient ratio, it involves considering individual factors, dietary preferences, and health goals. It's essential to prioritize nutrient-dense whole foods, including a variety of lean proteins, complex carbohydrates, and healthy fats, while limiting intake of processed and sugary foods. Consulting with a registered dietitian or nutritionist can provide personalized guidance and support in developing a balanced and sustainable eating plan tailored to individual needs.

Chapter three

Planning your meals

Meal planning is a systematic approach to organizing meals for a set period, typically a week, to ensure balanced nutrition, save time, and reduce food waste. Here's an exhaustive guide to meal planning:

1. Assess Your Needs: Consider dietary restrictions, preferences, and nutritional goals for yourself and your family members. Take into account factors like age, activity level, and any health conditions.

2. Set a Schedule: Decide how often you'll plan meals, whether it's weekly, bi-weekly, or monthly. Choose a day for planning and grocery shopping.

3. Create a Menu: Outline meals for each day, including breakfast, lunch, dinner, and snacks. Variety is key to prevent monotony and ensure balanced nutrition.

4. Balance Macronutrients: Aim for a balanced ratio of carbohydrates, proteins, and fats in each meal.Make sure your diet is rich in whole grains, fruits, veggies, lean meats, and healthy fats.

5. Consider Portion Sizes: Adjust portion sizes according to individual needs and calorie requirements. Use tools like measuring cups, scales, or visual cues to estimate portion sizes accurately.

6. Plan for Leftovers: Incorporate leftovers into your meal plan to minimize food waste and save time . Cook extra portions or repurpose ingredients into new dishes.

7. Use Seasonal Ingredients: Plan meals around seasonal produce to ensure freshness, flavor, and cost-effectiveness. Consider visiting farmers' markets or joining a community-supported agriculture (CSA) program.

8. Include Convenience Foods: Utilize pre-cut vegetables, canned beans, frozen fruits, and other convenience foods to streamline meal preparation, especially on busy days.

9. Batch Cooking: Dedicate a day for batch cooking staples like grains, proteins, and sauces to simplify meal assembly throughout the week.

10. Plan for Flexibility: Leave room for spontaneity by incorporating "flex meals" or theme nights like Taco Tuesday or Meatless Monday. Adapt recipes based on ingredient availability and preferences.

11. Check Inventory: Take inventory of pantry staples, freezer items, and perishables before creating your meal plan. Use up ingredients that are nearing expiration to minimize waste.

12. Shop Smart: Make a detailed grocery list based on your meal plan to avoid impulse purchases and ensure you have all the necessary ingredients. Consider shopping online for convenience and to compare prices.

13. Prep Ahead: Prepare ingredients in advance, such as washing and chopping vegetables, marinating meats, or pre-cooking grains, to streamline meal preparation during the week.

14. Stay Organized: Keep track of your meal plan, grocery lists, and recipes in a

centralized location, whether it's a physical planner, app, or spreadsheet. This helps you stay organized and stick to your plan.

15. Evaluate and Adjust: Reflect on your meal plan regularly to assess what worked well and what could be improved. Adjust your approach based on feedback from family members and changes in dietary needs or preferences.

By following these steps, you can create a comprehensive meal plan that meets your nutritional needs, saves time and money, and reduces stress associated with mealtime decision-making.

Meal prepping strategies

Meal prepping is a practical approach to streamline your cooking process, save time, money, and promote healthier eating habits. Here's an in-depth look at various strategies to effectively meal prep:

1. Planning: Start by planning your meals for the week ahead. Consider your dietary goals, preferences, and schedule. Make a list of recipes, ingredients, and portion sizes needed for each meal.

2. Batch Cooking: Prepare large batches of staple foods like grains, proteins, and vegetables. This allows you to cook once and enjoy multiple meals throughout the week. Examples include rice, quinoa, grilled chicken, and roasted vegetables.

3. Versatile Ingredients: Choose versatile ingredients that can be used in multiple dishes. For example, roasted vegetables can be added to salads, wraps, or grain bowls, providing variety without much extra effort.

4. Storage Containers: Invest in high-quality storage containers in various sizes to store prepped ingredients and meals. Opt for containers that are microwave-safe, stackable, and leak-proof to keep food fresh and easily accessible.

5. Portion Control: Use portion control tools like measuring cups, scales, or pre-portioned containers to ensure balanced meals and avoid overeating. This is particularly useful for those watching their calorie intake or trying to manage portion sizes.

6. Freezing Meals: Certain meals can freezing soups, stews, casseroles, and

sauces are great options. For simple identification, label containers with the contents and the date prepared in advance and frozen for later use.

7. Pre-cut and Washed Produce: Save time by prepping fruits and vegetables in advance. Wash,peel, chop, and store them in containers for quick and easy access when assembling meals or snacks.

8. Pre-portioned Snacks: Portion out snacks like nuts, seeds, fruits, and yogurt into grab-and-go containers or bags. This prevents mindless snacking and helps you stick to your dietary goals.

9. Theme Nights: Assign theme nights to your meal prep routine, such as Meatless Monday, Taco Tuesday, or Stir-Fry Friday. This adds variety to your meals while simplifying the planning process.

10.Prep in Stages: Break down meal prep into manageable stages throughout the week. For example, chop vegetables one day, cook proteins another day, and assemble meals the night before. This prevents burnout and makes the process more manageable.

11. Utilize Appliances: Take advantage of kitchen appliances like slow cookers, pressure cookers, and air fryers to streamline meal prep. These tools can help you cook large batches of food with minimal effort and supervision.

12. Leftover Transformation: Get creative with leftovers by repurposing them into new dishes. For example, use leftover roasted vegetables to make a frittata or add cooked grains to salads for extra texture and nutrients.

13. Family Involvement: Get the whole family involved in meal prep to share the workload and teach valuable cooking skills. Assign age-appropriate tasks like washing produce, stirring ingredients, or assembling meals.

14. Stay Organized: Keep your kitchen organized and clutter-free to streamline meal prep. Designate specific areas for prepping, cooking, and storing ingredients to avoid confusion and save time.

15. Review and Adapt: Periodically review your meal prep routine to identify what's working well and what could be improved. Be open to making adjustments based on

your changing needs, preferences, and schedule.

By incorporating these meal prepping strategies into your routine, you can simplify the cooking process, save time, and enjoy delicious and nutritious meals throughout the week.

Balancing macronutrients in every meal

Balancing macronutrients in every meal is essential for maintaining overall health, supporting energy levels, promoting satiety, and achieving fitness goals. Carbohydrates, proteins, and lipids are examples of macronutrients, often known as macros. Each of these macronutrients plays a distinct role in the body, and consuming them in appropriate proportions can help optimize nutrition and enhance well-being.

Understanding Macronutrients:

1. Carbohydrates: The body uses carbohydrates as its main energy source. They supply glucose, which powers our cells—especially those in the muscles and brain are the body's primary source of energy. They Carbohydrates can be found

in foods like grains, fruits, vegetables, and legumes.

2. Proteins: Proteins are crucial for building and repairing tissues, synthesizing hormones and enzymes, and supporting immune function. Dietary protein sources include meat, poultry, fish, eggs, dairy, tofu, legumes, and nuts.

3.   Fats: Fats are essential for hormone production, absorbing fat-soluble vitamins (A, D, E, K), providing insulation, and maintaining cell structure. Healthy fat sources include avocados, nuts, seeds, olive oil, fatty fish, and coconut oil.

Importance of Balanced Macronutrients:

Balancing macronutrients in each meal offers several benefits:

1. Sustained Energy: Including a combination of carbohydrates, proteins, and fats in every meal helps regulate blood sugar levels, providing a steady supply of energy throughout the day.

2. Enhanced Satiety: Consuming balanced meals promotes feelings of fullness and satisfaction, reducing the likelihood of

overeating or snacking on unhealthy foods between meals.

3. Improved Nutrient Absorption: Pairing macronutrients optimizes the absorption of essential vitamins and minerals, ensuring that the body can utilize nutrients effectively.

4. Support for Fitness Goals: Depending on individual fitness objectives, adjusting macronutrient ratios can aid in muscle growth, fat loss, or overall performance.

Strategies for Balancing Macronutrients:

1. Portion Control: Begin by understanding appropriate portion sizes for each macronutrient. For example, a balanced plate might consist of 1/2 vegetables (carbohydrates), 1/4 lean protein, and 1/4 healthy fats.

2. Include Whole Foods: Focus on whole, minimally processed foods to ensure a diverse intake of nutrientsThroughout your meals, include entire grains, lean meats, vibrant fruits and veggies, and healthy fats.

3. Choose Complex Carbohydrates: Opt for complex carbohydrates such as whole grains, sweet potatoes, quinoa, and legumes over refined carbohydrates like

white bread and sugary snacks. Complex carbs provide sustained energy and are rich in fiber and nutrients.

4. Prioritize Lean Proteins: Select lean sources of protein to minimize saturated fat intake. Examples include skinless poultry, fish, tofu, tempeh, beans, and low-fat dairy products.

5. Include Healthy Fats: Incorporate sources of healthy fats such as avocados, nuts, seeds, olive oil, and fatty fish into your meals. These fats support heart health and provide satiety.

6. Balance Ratios: While individual macronutrient needs vary based on factors like age, gender, activity level, and goals, a general guideline is to aim for a balanced ratio of approximately 40-60% carbohydrates, 20-30% protein, and 20-30% fat in each meal.

7. Consider Timing: Distribute macronutrients evenly throughout the day to maintain energy levels and support metabolism. Aim for balanced meals and snacks every 3-4 hours.

Practical Examples of Balanced Meals:

1. Breakfast:
   - Scrambled eggs with spinach and tomatoes (protein and vegetables)
   - Whole-grain toast (complex carbohydrates)
   - Avocado slices (healthy fats)

2. Lunch:
   - Grilled chicken breast (protein)
   - Quinoa salad with mixed vegetables (carbohydrates and fiber)
   - Olive oil vinaigrette dressing (healthy fats)

3. Dinner:
   - Baked salmon fillet (protein and omega-3 fats)
   - Steamed broccoli and carrots (carbohydrates and fiber)
   - Brown rice pilaf (complex carbohydrates)

4. Snack:
   - Greek yogurt with berries (protein and carbohydrates)
   - Handful of almonds (healthy fats).

Chapter Four

Protein Rich Recipes

Break fast

some protein-rich breakfast recipes:

1. Greek Yogurt Parfait: Layer Greek yogurt with mixed berries, nuts, and a drizzle of honey for a delicious and protein-packed breakfast.

2. Egg Muffins: Whisk together eggs, spinach, bell peppers, and cheese, then bake in muffin tins for convenient grab-and-go protein breakfasts.

3. Quinoa Breakfast Bowl: Cook quinoa and top it with sautéed vegetables, avocado, and a poached egg for a hearty and protein-rich breakfast.

4. Protein Pancakes: Use protein powder in your pancake batter, and serve with Greek yogurt and fruit for an extra protein boost.

5. Chia Seed Pudding: Mix chia seeds with almond milk and a scoop of protein powder, then let it sit overnight. Top with nuts and berries in the morning for a protein-packed breakfast.

6. Tofu Scramble: Sauté tofu with vegetables like mushrooms, onions, and spinach, seasoned with turmeric, garlic, and nutritional yeast for a tasty vegan protein breakfast option.

7. Protein Smoothie: Blend together protein powder, spinach, banana, almond milk, and nut butter for a quick and nutritious breakfast on the go.

8. Cottage Cheese Bowl: Top cottage cheese with sliced fruits, nuts, and a drizzle of honey for a simple yet satisfying protein-rich breakfast option.
Of course, here are some more protein-rich breakfast recipes:

9. Protein Oatmeal: Cook oats with milk or water, then stir in protein powder, nut butter, and sliced bananas for a filling and nutritious breakfast.

10. Salmon and Avocado Toast: Spread mashed avocado on whole grain toast and

top with smoked salmon and a sprinkle of chia seeds for a breakfast rich in healthy fats and protein.

11. Protein Waffles: Make waffles using protein powder in the batter and serve with Greek yogurt and fresh berries for a delicious and protein-packed breakfast option.

12. Breakfast Burrito: Fill a whole grain tortilla with scrambled eggs, black beans, diced tomatoes, avocado, and salsa for a protein-rich and flavorful breakfast wrap.

13. Soy Milk Smoothie Bowl: Blend together soy milk, frozen berries, tofu, and a scoop of protein powder, then top with granola, nuts, and seeds for a protein-packed breakfast bowl.

14. Egg and Veggie Breakfast Quesadilla: Fill a whole grain tortilla with scrambled eggs, sautéed vegetables, and cheese, then fold it over and cook until crispy for a protein-rich and satisfying breakfast.

15. Protein Breakfast Cookies: Bake cookies using protein powder, oats, nut butter, and mashed banana for a portable and protein-packed breakfast option.

16. Turkey and Cheese Breakfast Sandwich: Layer sliced turkey, cheese, and avocado between whole grain English muffins or bread for a protein-rich breakfast sandwich that's perfect for busy mornings.

17. Protein Power Bowl: Combine cooked quinoa, roasted sweet potatoes, black beans, avocado, and a fried egg for a nutrient-dense and protein-packed breakfast bowl.

18. Protein-Packed Chia Seed Pancakes: Make pancakes using chia seeds, oats, Greek yogurt, and eggs for a hearty and protein-rich breakfast option that's also gluten-free.

These recipes should help you start your day with a delicious and protein-packed breakfast!

Lunch

 some protein-rich lunch recipes you might enjoy:

1. Grilled Chicken Salad: Grilled chicken breast slices on a bed of mixed greens, topped with cherry tomatoes, cucumbers, avocado, and a light vinaigrette dressing.

2. Quinoa and Black Bean Bowl: Cooked quinoa mixed with black beans, corn, diced bell peppers, and diced avocado. Season with lime juice, cumin, and cilantro for extra flavor.

3. Lentil Soup: A hearty soup made with lentils, vegetables (like carrots, celery, and onions), and vegetable broth. You can add some diced chicken or turkey sausage for extra protein.

4. Tofu Stir-Fry: Cubes of tofu stir-fried with colorful vegetables such as bell peppers, broccoli, and snap peas, seasoned with soy sauce, garlic, and ginger.

5. Turkey and Veggie Wrap: Whole wheat tortilla filled with sliced turkey breast,

spinach leaves, shredded carrots, and
hummus or Greek yogurt spread.

6. Chickpea Salad: Chickpeas mixed with
diced cucumbers, tomatoes, red onions,
and parsley, dressed with lemon juice, olive
oil, and a sprinkle of feta cheese.

7. Salmon Quinoa Bowl: Baked or grilled
salmon served over cooked quinoa with
roasted vegetables like sweet potatoes,
Brussels sprouts, and asparagus.

8. Egg Salad Sandwich: Hard-boiled eggs
mashed with Greek yogurt or avocado,
mixed with diced celery, red onion, and
mustard, served on whole grain bread or
lettuce leaves.

9. Greek Yogurt Parfait: Layer Greek yogurt
with mixed berries, sliced bananas, and
granola for a protein-packed and satisfying
lunch option.

10. Beef and Broccoli Stir-Fry: Thinly sliced
beef sautéed with broccoli florets and garlic
in a soy sauce-based sauce, served over
brown rice or cauliflower rice.

11. Cottage Cheese and Fruit Plate:
Cottage cheese paired with fresh fruit slices
such as pineapple, strawberries, and kiwi,

sprinkled with almonds or walnuts for added crunch.

12. Tuna Salad Lettuce Wraps: Canned tuna mixed with diced celery, red onion, and avocado, seasoned with lemon juice and Dijon mustard, wrapped in lettuce leaves for a low-carb option.

13. Bean and Veggie Burrito Bowl: Cooked black beans or kidney beans served with sautéed bell peppers, onions, and corn, topped with salsa, avocado slices, and a sprinkle of cheese.

14. Chicken and Quinoa Stuffed Bell Peppers: Bell peppers stuffed with a mixture of cooked quinoa, shredded chicken breast, diced tomatoes, and black beans, baked until tender.

15. Shrimp and Avocado Salad: Grilled or sautéed shrimp served over mixed greens with sliced avocado, cherry tomatoes, and cucumber, dressed with a light citrus vinaigrette.

These protein-rich lunch ideas offer a variety of flavors and textures to keep your meals exciting and satisfying.

Dinner

some protein-rich dinner recipes:

1. Grilled Chicken Breast with Quinoa
Salad:
   - Marinate chicken breasts with olive oil,
lemon juice, garlic, and herbs.
   - Grill until cooked through.
   - Serve with a quinoa salad mixed with
chopped vegetables like cucumber,
tomatoes, bell peppers, and a sprinkle of
feta cheese.

2. Lentil and Vegetable Stir-Fry:
   - Sauté onions, garlic, and your choice of
vegetables (such as bell peppers, broccoli,
and carrots) in a pan.
   - Add cooked lentils and stir-fry sauce
(soy sauce, ginger, and a bit of honey or
maple syrup).
   - Serve with quinoa or brown rice.

3. Baked Salmon with Roasted Vegetables:
   - Lemon zest, salt, and pepper are used to
season salmon fillets.
   - Bake in the oven until cooked through.
   - Roast a mix of vegetables like sweet
potatoes, Brussels sprouts, and cauliflower
with olive oil and spices until tender.

- Roasted veggies should be used when serving the salmon

4. Tofu and Vegetable Stir-Fry:
   - Marinate tofu cubes in soy sauce, garlic, and ginger.
   - Sauté tofu in a pan until golden brown.
   - Add sliced vegetables like bell peppers, snap peas, and mushrooms, and cook until tender.
   - Serve with brown rice or noodles.

5. Chickpea and Spinach Curry:
   -Sauté onions, garlic, and ginger in a pot.
   - Add curry powder, cumin, coriander, and turmeric.
   - Add the coconut milk and canned beans and stir.

   - Add fresh spinach and cook until wilted.
   - Serve over basmati rice.

6. Beef and Broccoli Stir-Fry:
   - Slice beef thinly and marinate in soy sauce, garlic, and ginger.
   - Stir-fry beef in a hot pan until browned, then remove from the pan.
   - Add broccoli florets and sliced bell peppers to the same pan and cook until tender-crisp.

- Return the beef to the pan, add a splash of oyster sauce and sesame oil, and toss everything together.
   - Serve over brown rice or noodles.

7. Quinoa Stuffed Bell Peppers:- Prepare quinoa as directed on the package.
Cut bell peppers in half, then take out the membranes and seeds.
- Mix cooked quinoa with black beans, corn, diced tomatoes, diced onions, and spices like cumin and chili powder.
   - Stuff the mixture into the bell pepper halves and bake until peppers are tender.
   - Optionally, top with shredded cheese before baking.

8. Turkey and Veggie Skewers:
   - Thread chunks of turkey breast, cherry tomatoes, zucchini slices, and bell pepper onto skewers.
   - Brush with olive oil and season with salt, pepper, and your favorite herbs (such as thyme or rosemary).
   - Grill or bake until turkey is cooked through and veggies are tender.
   - Accompany with a green salad or quinoa side dish.

9. Eggplant and Chickpea Tagine:
   - Sauté onions, garlic, and diced eggplant in a tagine or large pot until softened.

- Add canned chickpeas, diced tomatoes, vegetable broth, and Moroccan spices like cumin, paprika, and cinnamon.
  - Simmer until flavors meld and eggplant is tender.

  - Serve over couscous and garnish with chopped fresh cilantro or parsley.

10. Shrimp and Avocado Salad:
  - Grill or sauté shrimp seasoned with salt, pepper, and garlic until cooked through.
  - Toss together mixed greens, sliced avocado, cherry tomatoes, and cucumber.
  - Top with the cooked shrimp and drizzle with a simple dressing made with olive oil, lemon juice, and Dijon mustard.

These recipes offer delicious and nutritious options to enjoy a protein-rich dinner.

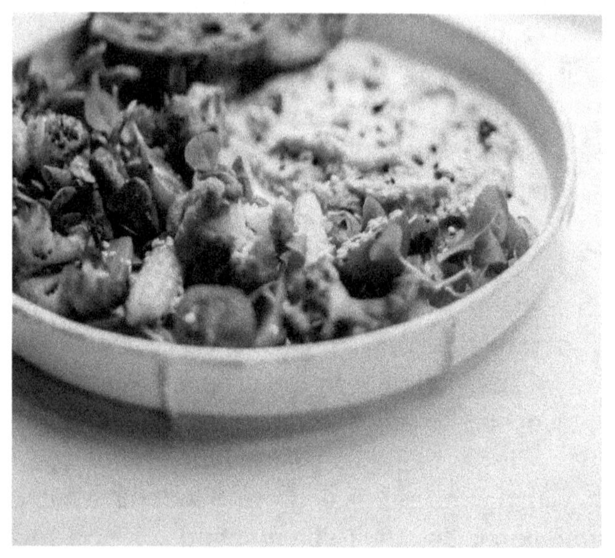

Chapter Five

Fat Rich Recipes

Breakfast

some hearty and indulgent breakfast recipes:

1. Avocado Bacon Breakfast Sandwich: Layer crispy bacon, sliced avocado, and a fried egg between two slices of toasted bread or English muffins. Add some cheese or mayo for extra richness.

2. Banana Nutella Stuffed French Toast: Spread Nutella on slices of bread, sandwich sliced bananas between them, dip in a mixture of beaten eggs and milk, and fry until golden brown. Serve with a drizzle of Nutella on top.

3. Loaded Breakfast Burrito: Fill a large tortilla with scrambled eggs, cooked sausage or bacon, shredded cheese, diced potatoes, and salsa. Roll it up and enjoy!

4. Creamy Mushroom and Spinach Omelette: Sautee mushrooms and spinach until tender, then pour beaten eggs over the top. Cook until set, fold in half, and sprinkle with cheese before serving.

5. Chocolate Chip Pancakes: Add chocolate chips to your pancake batter before cooking. Top with whipped cream and maple syrup for a decadent treat.

6. Eggs Benedict: Toast English muffins, top with Canadian bacon or smoked salmon, poached eggs, and hollandaise sauce. Add some fresh herbs, such parsley or chives, as a garnish.

7. Sausage Gravy and Biscuits: Serve warm buttermilk biscuits topped with a creamy sausage gravy made from cooked sausage, flour, milk, and seasoning.

8. Cinnamon Roll Waffles: Place refrigerated cinnamon roll dough in a preheated waffle iron and cook until golden brown and crispy. Drizzle with icing and

sprinkle with chopped nuts or powdered
sugar.

9. Cheesy Breakfast Hashbrown Casserole:
Mix shredded hash browns with cooked
breakfast sausage, diced bell peppers,
onions, and plenty of shredded cheese.
Bake until bubbly and golden brown.

10. Ricotta Pancakes with Berry
Compote:Make fluffy pancakes using ricotta
cheese in the batter. Serve with a warm
berry compote made by simmering mixed
berries with a bit of sugar and lemon juice
until thickened.
These recipes are sure to make your
breakfasts extra special and satisfying!

Lunch

few recipes for a rich and satisfying lunch:

1. Creamy Mushroom Risotto: Cook Arborio
rice in vegetable broth with sautéed
mushrooms, onions, garlic, and a splash of
white wine. Finish with heavy cream and
parmesan cheese for a luxurious texture.

2. Beef Stroganoff: Sauté beef strips with
onions and garlic, then simmer in a rich
sauce made with beef broth, sour cream,

and a touch of mustard. Serve over egg noodles or rice.

3. Chicken Alfredo Pasta: Cook fettuccine according to package instructions. Meanwhile, sauté chicken breast in butter until cooked through, then add heavy cream and parmesan cheese to create a creamy Alfredo sauce. Toss with cooked pasta and garnish with parsley.

4. Loaded Baked Potato Soup: Simmer diced potatoes, onions, and garlic in chicken broth until tender. Mash some of the potatoes to thicken the soup, then stir in heavy cream, cheddar cheese, crispy bacon, and chopped green onions.

5. Grilled Cheese and Tomato Soup: Make a classic grilled cheese sandwich with thick slices of bread and a combination of your favorite cheeses. Serve alongside a rich, homemade tomato soup made with roasted tomatoes, onions, garlic, and cream.

6. Truffle Mac and Cheese: Cook macaroni pasta according to package instructions. Meanwhile, make a creamy cheese sauce with butter, flour, milk, and a combination of sharp cheddar and Gruyère cheese. Add a drizzle of truffle oil for extra indulgence before serving.

7.   Creamy Spinach and Artichoke Stuffed Chicken: Butterfly chicken breasts and stuff with a mixture of cream cheese, chopped spinach, marinated artichoke hearts, and grated Parmesan. Secure with toothpicks, then bake until golden and cooked through.

8. Lobster Bisque: Sauté onions, carrots, and celery in butter until soft. Add lobster stock, diced cooked lobster meat, and heavy cream.Blend till smooth after simmering to let flavors merge.Serve garnished with a drizzle of sherry and chopped chives.

9. Sausage and Peppers Pasta: Sauté sliced Italian sausage with bell peppers and onions until caramelized. Toss with cooked pasta and a creamy tomato sauce made with heavy cream, crushed tomatoes, garlic, and Italian herbs.

10. Creamy Bacon Carbonara: Cook spaghetti until al dente. Meanwhile, sauté diced bacon until crispy, then remove from the pan. In the same pan, whisk together eggs, heavy cream, grated Parmesan cheese, and black pepper. Toss cooked pasta with the sauce until coated, then stir in the crispy bacon.

These recipes should provide you with plenty of rich and satisfying lunch options.

Dinner

Here are a couple of dinner recipes that are rich in flavor but can be made healthier by using leaner cuts of meat or incorporating more vegetables:

1. Grilled Salmon with Avocado Salsa:Marinate salmon fillets in a mixture of lemon juice, olive oil, garlic, and herbs. Grill until cooked through. Meanwhile, make a salsa by combining diced avocado, tomato, red onion, cilantro, lime juice, salt, and pepper. Serve the grilled salmon topped with the avocado salsa.

2. Mushroom Risotto: Sauté chopped onions and garlic in olive oil until softened. Add Arborio rice and cook until lightly toasted. Gradually add chicken or vegetable broth, stirring frequently, until the rice is creamy and cooked through. Stir in sautéed mushrooms, Parmesan cheese, and a splash of white wine for extra richness.

3. Stuffed Bell Peppers: Cut the tops off bell peppers and remove the seeds. In a skillet,

cook ground turkey or lean ground beef with diced onions, garlic, and your favorite spices until browned. Place the mixture inside the bell peppers and sprinkle additional cheese on top. Bake until the cheese is bubbling and melted and the peppers are soft.
 Stir in cooked rice, black beans, diced tomatoes, corn, and a handful of shredded cheese.

4. Vegetable Coconut Curry: In a large pot, sauté diced onions, garlic, ginger, and curry paste in coconut oil until fragrant. Add diced sweet potatoes, carrots, bell peppers, and any other vegetables of your choice. Pour in coconut milk and vegetable broth, then simmer until the vegetables are tender. Serve over cooked quinoa or brown rice, garnished with fresh cilantro and lime wedges.

5. Creamy Tuscan Chicken: In a skillet, brown seasoned chicken breasts in olive oil until cooked through. Remove the chicken and set aside. In the same skillet, sauté minced garlic, sun-dried tomatoes, and spinach until the spinach is wilted. Pour in heavy cream and chicken broth, then simmer until slightly thickened. the chicken should be returned to the skillet and simmer

when heated through. Serve over cooked
pasta or with crusty bread.

6.   Beef and Broccoli Stir-Fry: Thinly
slice beef steak and marinate in a mixture of
soy sauce, garlic, ginger, and a touch of
honey.

In a large skillet, stir-fry the marinated beef
until browned. Remove from the pan and
set aside. Stir-fry broccoli florets, sliced bell
peppers, and thinly sliced carrots until
tender-crisp. Return the beef to the pan and
toss everything together with a sauce made
from soy sauce, oyster sauce, and a splash
of sesame oil. Serve over steamed rice.

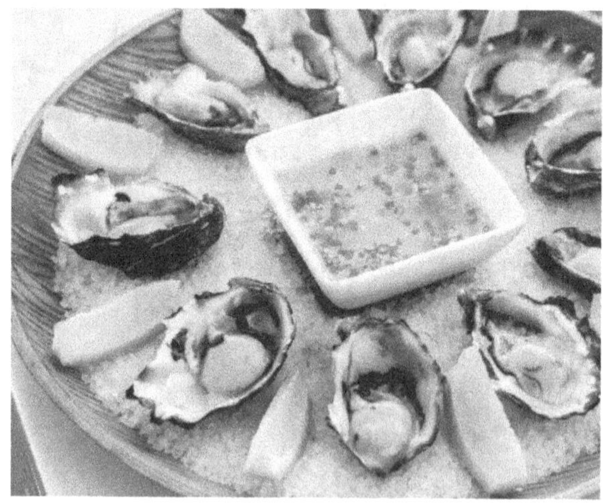

Oyster sauce

Chapter Six

Carbohydrate Rich Recipes

Breakfast

Breakfast is often touted as the most important meal of the day, providing us with the energy and nutrients needed to kick-start our morning and fuel our activities. For those seeking carbohydrate-rich options to power through their day, there are numerous delicious and nutritious recipes to explore.   These breakfast recipes is packed with carbohydrates, offering both traditional favorites and innovative twists to satisfy your taste buds and nutritional needs.

1. Oatmeal Delights
   - Oatmeal is a classic breakfast choice, rich in complex carbohydrates that provide sustained energy throughout the morning. Start with rolled oats or steel-cut oats for a hearty base.
   - Classic Oatmeal: Cook oats with water or milk until creamy, then top with fruits,

nuts, seeds, and a drizzle of honey or maple syrup for added sweetness and flavor.

   - Overnight Oats: Combine oats with your choice of liquid (milk, yogurt, or plant-based alternatives), along with toppings like chia seeds, sliced fruits, and a dash of cinnamon. Let it soak overnight for a convenient grab-and-go option in the morning.

   - Baked Oatmeal: Mix oats with eggs, milk, sweeteners, and flavorings, then bake until set for a nutritious and satisfying breakfast casserole.

2. Pancake Extravaganza:

   - Pancakes are a beloved breakfast treat, and with a few ingredient swaps, they can become a wholesome source of carbohydrates.

   - Banana Oat Pancakes: Blend ripe bananas with oats, eggs, and a splash of milk to create a batter that's both fluffy and nutritious. Cook on a griddle until golden brown, then serve with fresh fruit and a dollop of yogurt.

   - Whole Wheat Pancakes: For more nutrients and fiber, use whole wheat flour in place of all-purpose flour. Serve with pureed berries or a drizzle of homemade fruit compote for a burst of flavor.

   - Protein Pancakes: Amp up the protein content by adding Greek yogurt or protein powder to your pancake batter. Pair with sliced almonds and a sprinkle of ground flaxseeds for extra crunch and nutritional benefits.

3. Hearty Breakfast Bowls:

- Breakfast bowls offer a customizable way to incorporate a variety of nutrient-dense ingredients, including carbohydrates, proteins, and healthy fats.

- Acai Bowls: Blend frozen acai berries with bananas, berries, and a splash of liquid (such as coconut water or almond milk) to create a thick and creamy base. Top with granola, sliced fruits, coconut flakes, and a drizzle of honey for a refreshing and energizing breakfast option.

- Quinoa Breakfast Bowl: Cook quinoa in water or milk until fluffy, then top with roasted sweet potatoes, sautéed greens, avocado slices, and a poached egg for a balanced and filling meal.

- Muesli Bowls: Combine rolled oats with dried fruits, nuts, seeds, and yogurt for a Swiss-inspired breakfast bowl that's both nutritious and satisfying

For added taste, add a sprinkling of cinnamon or a drizzle of honey.

4. Energizing Smoothie Creations: An easy and quick method to get plenty of vitamins, minerals, and carbohydrates into your diet is with a smoothie.

- Tropical Paradise Smoothie: For a colorful and hydrating breakfast choice, blend frozen pineapple, mango, and banana with a little spinach and coconut water. For even more satisfaction, mix in a scoop of protein powder or Greek yogurt.

- Berry Blast Smoothie: For a high-fiber, high-antioxidant breakfast smoothie, combine mixed berries (strawberries, blueberries, and raspberries) with Greek yogurt, almond milk, and a scoop of oats. For added nutrients, personalize with a sprinkling of hemp seeds or a drizzle of almond butter.

- Green Goddess Smoothie: For a creamy, nutrient-dense breakfast smoothie, blend leafy greens (such spinach or kale) with avocado, banana, and a dash of orange juice. Increase the amount of carbohydrates by adding cooked sweet potatoes or oats for long-lasting energy in the morning.

These above mouthwatering and wholesome breakfast recipes will provide you the energy and vitality you need to tackle the day.

Lunch.

It can be difficult to find the time to cook a healthy lunch in the fast-paced world of today. But with the correct recipes and a little preparation, you can have a filling, tasty lunch that will provide you with plenty of carbs to go through the rest of the day. Carbohydrates are an integral part of every balanced diet since they are necessary nutrients that provide your body energy.

1. Roasted Vegetable and Quinoa Salad: - Ingredients:
One cup of quinoa, a variety of veggies (such as bell peppers, zucchini, and cherry tomatoes), and olive oil
- To taste, add salt and pepper - Optional fresh herbs
- Feta cheese, if desired
- Directions:
Set the oven's temperature to 400°F, or 200°C.

2. Cook the quinoa as directed on the package after giving it a quick rinse in cold water.
3. Dice the veggies into small pieces and combine them with salt, pepper, and olive oil.
4. Arrange the veggies on a baking sheet and bake for 20 to 25 minutes, or until they are soft and have a hint of caramel.
5. Combine the cooked quinoa and roasted veggies in a big bowl.
6. Drizzle with additional olive oil and, if like, top with feta cheese and fresh herbs.
7. Serve warm or room temperature after giving everything a gentle toss to mix.

Nutritional Advantages: Quinoa contains all nine necessary amino acids, making it a complete protein.
- Vegetables improve general health and digestive health by adding fiber, vitamins, and minerals to the meal.

2.   Quesadillas with Sweet Potato and Black Beans:

 - Ingredients:
One can of rinsed and drained black beans; two large sweet potatoes, peeled and chopped; one diced red onion
- Tacos made of whole wheat

- Shredded cheese, such as Mexican blend or cheddar
- To taste, add chili powder, paprika, and cumin; - Add fresh cilantro (optional)
1 Greek yogurt and salsa to serve

- Directions:
1. Boil or steam the sweet potatoes until they are soft. Once drained, use a fork to mash.

Diced onion should be sautéed in a skillet until transparent. Incorporate the spices, mashed sweet potatoes, and black beans. Cook until well heated.
3. Lay out a tortilla on a flat surface, then cover half of it with the sweet potato and black bean mixture.
4. Fold the tortilla in half and top with cheese that has been shredded.
5. Continue with the remaining filling and tortillas.
6. Place the quesadillas in a big skillet over medium heat and cook them for two to three minutes on each side, or until crispy and golden.
7. Cut into wedges, top with freshly chopped cilantro, and serve with Greek yogurt and salsa on the side.

Nutritional Advantages: - Sweet potatoes are high in fiber, vitamins A and C, and complex carbs.
- Black beans help with weight management by providing satiety and fiber along with protein.

3.   Asian Chickpea Wrap: -

Containments:
- Pitas or whole wheat wraps
- Drained and washed chickpeas from one can - Halved cherry tomatoes - Diced cucumber
- Sliced red onion thinly - Pitted and halved Kalamata olives - Feta cheese crumbles
- Chopped fresh parsley - Tzatziki and hummus for spreading

- Directions:
1. Combine the chickpeas, cucumber, red onion, olives, parsley, and cherry tomatoes in a bowl.
2. Use a skillet or microwave to reheat the wraps or pitas.
3. Top each wrap or pita with a layer of hummus and tzatziki sauce.
4. Place a spoonful of the chickpea mixture in the middle of each pita or wrap.
5. Top with feta cheese crumbles.
6. Tightly coil up, folding in the sides and, if needed, secure with a toothpick.

7. Cut in half on the diagonal and serve right away.

Nutritional Advantages: - Chickpeas are a great source of fiber and plant-based protein, which helps with digestion and supports heart health.
- Nutrients and healthy fats included in Mediterranean foods, such as feta cheese and olives, support general health.

incorporating meals high in carbohydrates into your lunchtime routine is an easy and efficient method to promote your general health and increase your energy levels.

Dinner

A balanced diet must include carbohydrates since they provide you energy and important nutrients. Including a choice of foods high in carbohydrates in your supper recipes will not only increase the satisfaction factor of your meals but also offer a variety of nutrients. We'll look at tasty and healthful meal ideas with a range of carbohydrates, such as grains, veggies, and legumes, in this collection of recipes.

1. Mediterranean Quinoa Salad: cooked quinoa combined with chopped red onion, cucumbers, cherry tomatoes, and crumbled feta cheese. tossed in a vinaigrette consisting of lemon juice, olive oil, oregano, and garlic. Serve as a cool and light dinner alternative that is ideal for summertime.

2. Enchiladas with Sweet Potato and Black Beans- Soft corn tortillas stuffed with black beans, corn, sliced bell peppers, and onions along with mashed sweet potatoes.
- Rolled up and covered with cheese shreds and enchilada sauce.
- Baked till bubbling and presented with sliced avocado and a dollop of Greek yogurt.

3. Spaghetti Aglio e Olio: Al dente spaghetti is combined with olive oil, garlic, red pepper flakes, and parsley to make a sauce. concluded with a squeeze of fresh lemon juice and a dusting of Parmesan cheese. This spaghetti meal, which is tasty but simple, is ideal for hectic weeknights.

4. Quinoa and Chickpea filled Bell Peppers - Cooked quinoa, cooked chickpeas, chopped tomatoes, spinach, and seasonings are filled inside hollowed-out bell peppers.

Baked until the filling is heated through and the peppers are soft. - For extra taste, serve with tangy tzatziki sauce on the side.

5. Vegetable Fried Rice - Soy sauce, ginger, garlic, and sesame oil are used to flavor cooked jasmine rice that is stir-fried with a variety of vegetables, including broccoli, carrots, peas, and bell peppers.
- Add some sliced green onions as a garnish, and this dish makes a filling and substantial supper.

Creamy risotto cooked with Arborio rice, roasted butternut squash, fresh sage, and vegetable broth is called Butternut Squash and Sage Risotto.
- completed with a balsamic glaze drizzle and a dusting of grated Parmesan cheese. This hearty recipe is ideal for cold nights spent at home.

7. Chickpea Tikka Masala - Chickpeas cooked with onions, garlic, ginger, and a mixture of Indian spices in a tasty tomato-based sauce. Transfer to warmed basmati rice and sprinkle with chopped fresh cilantro. This vegetarian version of a traditional Indian meal will definitely quench your thirst for strong flavors.
8. Caprese Quinoa Stuffed Peppers - Baked until the peppers are soft and the stuffing is

well heated, bell peppers filled with cooked quinoa, diced tomatoes, fresh mozzarella cheese, and chopped basil. - Drizzled with balsamic glaze.
- Serve as a healthy and light supper alternative that is ideal for summertime nights.

9. Lentil Shepherd's Pie - A flavorful gravy with cooked lentils combined with sliced carrots, onions, and celery. layered with smooth mashed potatoes on top, then baked till golden brown. This filling dish is ideal for chilly winter evenings.

10. Zucchini Noodles with Pesto and Cherry Tomatoes - Homemade basil pesto is combined with spiralized zucchini noodles, and cherry tomatoes are cut in half.
- Add pine nuts and freshly grated Parmesan cheese as garnishes. This fresh, flavorful, low-carb take on traditional spaghetti is light and fluffy.

 adding foods high in carbohydrates to your supper recipes is a tasty method to delight your palate and feed your body. There are lots of options to pick from, whether you like robust grains, savory veggies, or protein-rich legumes. Try varying the tastes and ingredients to make wholesome, filling meals that you'll enjoy eating.

Chapter Seven

Treats & Snacks

protein-based munchies

There's a solid reason why protein snacks and sweets have grown in popularity in recent years. They offer a tasty and enjoyable approach to sate cravings while supporting your health and fitness goals, in addition to being a practical way to increase your protein intake. There are many options to fit every taste and dietary requirement, ranging from handmade energy balls to protein bars.

 Advantages of Treats and Snacks with Protein:

1. Muscle Growth and Repair: Protein is a necessary food for everyone who engages in regular exercise or physical activity since it is necessary for muscle growth and repair. Snacking on high-protein foods throughout the day can promote muscle growth and

repair, speeding up the recovery process following exercise.

2. Fullness: Because protein is known to keep you feeling full and content, it can improve weight management efforts by preventing overeating. You may prevent cravings and avoid hunger pangs by including high-protein snacks in your diet in between meals.

3. Surge in Energy: Protein is a great option for a pre- or post-workout snack since it offers a consistent source of energy. Protein snacks may help you stay energized and focused, whether you need a little pick-me-up before working out or some fuel to recover afterward.

4. Nutrient Density: A lot of protein snacks and treats are rich in protein as well as other vital nutrients including minerals, vitamins, and good fats. Their high nutrient density renders them an advantageous supplement to your diet, offering several health advantages in addition to protein.

Variety of Protein Treats and Snacks:

1. Protein Bars: Available in a variety of flavors and formulations, protein bars are arguably the most popular type of protein

snack. They are easy to carry with you for on-the-go snacking, and they usually contain a combination of fats, carbohydrates, and protein sources like soy, whey, or pea protein.

2. Cookies with proteins: Protein cookies are a delicious substitute for regular cookies, consisting of components such as nut butter, oats, and protein powder. Depending on your taste, they can be crispy or soft and chewy, and they frequently have less sugar than their traditional cousins.

3. Bites/Protein Balls: These little sweets are ideal for sating desires without throwing off your well-laid diet. Made with components like protein powder, almonds, and dates, they are simple to flavor and keep in the freezer or refrigerator for a convenient on-the-go snack.

4 Waffles/pancakes with protein: Who says waffles and pancakes can't be nutritious? You can increase the protein content of these beloved breakfast recipes without sacrificing their fluffy texture and mouthwatering flavor by mixing protein powder into the batter.

5. Smoothies with Protein: Protein smoothies are a tasty and easy method to meet your daily protein needs, even while they aren't exactly snacks or treats in and of themselves. To make a wholesome and filling drink, simply blend together your preferred protein powder, fruits, veggies, and other ingredients.

Innovative Recipes for Protein Snacks and Treats:

1. Protein Bars with Peanut Butter:
Ingredients: - 1/2 cup peanut butter - 1 cup rolled oats
- 1/4 cup of protein powder; - 1/4 cup of honey or maple syrup
- 1/4 cup of optionally chopped nuts or seeds
- Guidelines:
1. Put the protein powder, chopped nuts or seeds, and oats (if using) in a big mixing bowl.
2. Melt the peanut butter and honey/maple syrup in the microwave in a another bowl, then whisk until smooth.
3. Drizzle the dry ingredients with the peanut butter mixture and stir until thoroughly blended.
4. To set, press the mixture into a baking dish that has been lined and chill for at least an hour.

5. Cut into bars and refrigerate for up to a week after the mixture has hardened.

2. Protein Cookies with Chocolate Chips:
Ingredients: - 1/4 cup protein powder - 1 cup almond flour
- One-fourth cup coconut sugar
- 1/4 cup melted coconut oil
- One egg
One-half teaspoon vanilla extract
1/4 cup chips made with dark chocolate
- Guidelines:
1. Preheat the oven to 350°F (175°C) and place parchment paper on a baking pan.
2. Combine almond flour, protein powder, and coconut sugar in a sizable mixing dish.
3. Beat the egg, vanilla extract, and melted coconut oil in a another bowl.
4. Combine the wet and dry components, mixing them thoroughly.
5. Add the chocolate chips and fold.
6. Place dough spoonfuls onto the baking sheet that has been prepared, then gently press them down with a fork.
7. Bake for ten to twelve minutes, or until the edges are browned.
8. Let cool for a few minutes on the baking sheet, then move to a wire rack to finish cooling.

3. Protein Balls Without Baking:

Ingredients: - 1/2 cup almond butter - 1 cup rolled oats
- 1/4 cup maple syrup or honey
- One-fourth cup protein powder
1/4 cup chips made with dark chocolate
One teaspoon of vanilla extract

- Guidelines:

1. Combine chocolate chips, protein powder, and oats in a large mixing dish.

2. Melt the almond butter and honey/maple syrup in the microwave in a another bowl, and then mix in the vanilla extract.

3. Drizzle the dry ingredients with the almond butter mixture and stir until thoroughly blended.

4. Using your hands, roll the mixture into balls and arrange them on a baking sheet covered with parchment paper.
5. To set before serving, place in the refrigerator for at least 30 minutes.

Protein snacks and treats are a tasty and practical method to increase your protein intake, satisfy cravings, and help you reach your fitness and health objectives. There are lots of delicious options to try, whether you prefer store-bought or handmade meals. You may gain from higher muscle growth and repair, better overall nutrition, increased satiety, and sustained energy levels by include protein-rich snacks in your diet. So feel free to treat yourself to a protein-rich treat today.

Snacks with carbs

Carbohydrates: Your Body's Fuel

Along with proteins and fats, carbohydrates, also known as "carbs," are one of the three macronutrients that are critical to human health. They are our body's main energy source, supplying the necessary fuel for a variety of internal processes, such as mental and physical activity. Carbohydrates are present in a broad variety of meals, from fruits and vegetables to grains and legumes, and they can take the form of sugars, starches, or fibers.
carbohydrate-rich snacks and sweets in this extensive guide, discussing their function in our diet, their effects on our health, and some delectable options to sate your desires while providing your body with nourishment.

Knowing Your Carbohydrates:

Atoms of carbon, hydrogen, and oxygen are combined in different ways to form carbohydrates. They fall into three primary categories:

1. Sugars: single- or double-molecule sugars make up simple carbohydrates. Examples are present in glucose, fructose, and sucrose.
naturally in fruits, honey, and dairy products, as well as added sugars in processed foods and beverages.

2. Starches: Complex carbohydrates made up of long chains of glucose molecules. Starches are abundant in foods like grains (wheat, rice, oats), legumes (beans, lentils), and starchy vegetables (potatoes, corn).

3. Fiber: Another type of complex carbohydrate, fiber is composed of indigestible plant material that provides numerous health benefits, including improved digestion, weight management, and reduced risk of chronic diseases. Fiber is found in fruits, vegetables, whole grains, nuts, and seeds.

The Role of Carbohydrates in the Body:

Carbohydrates serve as the primary source of energy for the body, particularly for high-intensity activities like exercise. When consumed, carbohydrates are broken down into glucose, which enters the bloodstream and is transported to cells to be used for energy. Excess glucose is stored in the liver and muscles as glycogen for future use.

In addition to providing energy, carbohydrates play a crucial role in brain function. The brain relies heavily on glucose as its primary fuel source, making carbohydrates essential for cognitive function and mental clarity.

Furthermore, carbohydrates contribute to the flavor, texture, and palatability of foods, making them an integral part of our diet from both a nutritional and culinary perspective.

The Importance of Choosing Healthy Carbohydrate Sources:

Not all carbohydrates are created equal. While some provide essential nutrients and health benefits, others offer little more than empty calories and can contribute to weight gain and chronic diseases like obesity, type 2 diabetes, and heart disease.

When selecting carbohydrate-rich snacks and treats, it's important to prioritize whole, minimally processed foods that are rich in nutrients and fiber. These include:

- Fruits: Fresh, whole fruits like apples, berries, and bananas are excellent sources of natural sugars, vitamins, minerals, and fiber. They make for convenient, portable snacks that satisfy your sweet tooth while nourishing your body.

- Vegetables: Non-starchy vegetables like carrots, cucumbers, and bell peppers are low in calories and high in fiber, making them ideal for snacking. Pair them with hummus or yogurt-based dips for added flavor and protein.

- Whole Grains: Choose whole grains like oats, quinoa, and brown rice over refined grains like white bread and pasta.The bran and germ of whole grains, which are high in fiber, vitamins, and minerals, are retained.Enjoy whole grain crackers, popcorn, or air-popped corn chips for a satisfying snack.

- Legumes: Beans, lentils, and chickpeas are nutritious plant-based sources of carbohydrates, protein, and fiber. Incorporate them into salads, soups, or homemade dips like hummus for a filling and flavorful snack.

- Nuts and Seeds: Rich in healthy fats, protein, and fiber, nuts and seeds make for satisfying and nutritious snacks. Enjoy a handful of almonds, walnuts, or pumpkin seeds for a crunchy and portable energy boost.

- Dairy: Opt for plain or low-sugar dairy products like Greek yogurt or cottage cheese, which provide a combination of carbohydrates, protein, and calcium. Add fresh fruit, nuts, or a drizzle of honey for natural sweetness and extra flavor.

Healthy Carbohydrate Snack Ideas:

Now that we understand the importance of choosing healthy carbohydrate sources, let's explore some delicious snack ideas that will keep you energized and satisfied throughout the day:

1. Fruit and Nut Butter: Spread almond or peanut butter on apple slices or banana

halves for a sweet and satisfying snack packed with fiber, healthy fats, and protein.

2. Greek Yogurt Parfait:Layer Greek yogurt with fresh berries, granola, and a drizzle of honey for a protein-rich snack that's perfect for breakfast or any time of day.

3. Veggie Sticks and Hummus: Dip carrot, cucumber, and bell pepper sticks into creamy hummus for a crunchy and nutritious snack loaded with fiber and plant-based protein.

4. Whole Grain Toast with Avocado: Top whole grain toast with mashed avocado, cherry tomatoes, and a sprinkle of sea salt for a savory and satisfying snack that's rich in fiber, healthy fats, and vitamins.

5. Trail Mix: Combine mixed nuts, dried fruits, and whole grain cereal for a portable and customizable snack that provides a balance of carbohydrates, protein, and healthy fats.

6. Homemade Energy Bites: Mix rolled oats, nut butter, honey, and dark chocolate chips to form bite-sized energy balls. Store them in the refrigerator for a convenient and delicious snack on the go.

7. Whole Grain Crackers with Cheese: Pair whole grain crackers with sliced cheese for a satisfying and protein-rich snack that's perfect for satisfying your cravings between meals.

Indulgent Carbohydrate Treats:

While it's important to prioritize nutrient-dense carbohydrate sources in our diet, it's also okay to enjoy indulgent treats in moderation. Here are some delicious carbohydrate-rich treats to satisfy your sweet tooth:

1. Dark Chocolate: Indulge in a square or two of dark chocolate (70% cocoa or higher) for a rich and satisfying treat that's loaded with antioxidants and flavonoids.

2. Homemade Banana Bread: Bake a loaf of moist and flavorful banana bread using whole wheat flour, ripe bananas, and a hint of cinnamon for a comforting and satisfying treat.

3. Oatmeal Cookies: Whip up a batch of chewy oatmeal cookies loaded with rolled oats, raisins, and chopped nuts for a wholesome and delicious snack that's perfect for sharing.

4. Fruit Sorbet: Blend frozen fruits like mangoes, berries, or pineapple with a splash of coconut water or fruit juice to create a refreshing and naturally sweet sorbet that's dairy-free and guilt-free.

5. Whole Grain Pancakes: Treat yourself to a stack of fluffy whole grain pancakes topped with fresh berries, maple syrup, and a dollop of Greek yogurt for a nutritious and indulgent breakfast or brunch option.

6. Sweet Potato Brownies: Bake fudgy brownies using sweet potato puree, cocoa powder, and whole grain flour for a decadent and nutrient-rich dessert that's sure to satisfy your chocolate cravings.

7. Fruit Crisp: Make a comforting fruit crisp using your favorite seasonal fruits topped with a crunchy oat and nut.

Fats Snacks

satisfying mouthfeel From velvety chocolate truffles to buttery croissants, from crispy bacon-wrapped dates to creamy cheesecakes, the world of fats snacks and treats offers a symphony of indulgence that can captivate even the most disciplined of palates.

The Seduction of Flavor:

At the heart of every fats snack and treat lies an explosion of flavor that titillates the taste buds and ignites the senses. From the deep, earthy notes of dark chocolate to the salty-sweet allure of caramel, each indulgence offers a symphony of tastes that dance across the palate with exquisite precision.

Consider, for instance, the humble potato chip. Crisp, salty, and utterly addictive, this iconic snack owes its irresistible flavor to the perfect balance of salt, fat, and umami-rich seasonings. With each satisfying crunch, the savory essence of the potato is elevated to new heights, leaving behind a lingering craving for just one more bite.

Similarly, the allure of a freshly baked cinnamon roll lies in its intoxicating aroma and decadent blend of spices. As the warm, buttery pastry unfurls with each bite, the mingling flavors of cinnamon, sugar, and vanilla envelop the senses in a blissful haze of indulgence.

The Art of Texture:

Beyond flavor, fats snacks and treats seduce the palate with their exquisite textures, ranging from crisp and crunchy to smooth and velvety. It is this interplay of textures that elevates these indulgences from mere sustenance to culinary works of art.

Consider the delicate flakiness of a perfectly baked croissant, its buttery layers yielding with a gentle crackle at the slightest touch. Each bite offers a symphony of textures, from the crisp exterior to the tender, airy crumb within, creating a sensory experience that is as satisfying to the touch as it is to the taste buds.

In contrast, the creamy richness of a decadent chocolate truffle melts effortlessly on the tongue, its velvety smoothness a testament to the skill of the chocolatier. With each luxurious bite, the chocolate envelops the palate in a silken embrace, leaving behind a lingering sensation of pure indulgence.

Yet, the allure of fats snacks and treats extends beyond mere sensory pleasure; it taps into the complex workings of the human psyche, offering comfort, nostalgia, and escape in equal measure. In a world fraught with stress and uncertainty, these indulgences serve as a temporary reprieve from the rigors of daily life, offering a moment of solace and pleasure in an otherwise chaotic world.

Consider the simple pleasure of a warm, gooey brownie enjoyed on a rainy day. As the rich chocolate melts in the mouth, it evokes memories of childhood, of simpler times filled with warmth and laughter. In that moment, the brownie becomes more than a mere confection; it becomes a source of comfort and reassurance, a tangible reminder of life's sweeter moments.

Similarly, the act of indulging in a decadent dessert with loved ones fosters a sense of connection and intimacy, strengthening bonds and creating lasting memories. Whether shared over a romantic dinner or enjoyed with friends on a lazy Sunday afternoon, these moments of indulgence serve to deepen relationships and cultivate a sense of belonging in an increasingly fragmented world.

In the world of culinary delights, fats snacks and treats occupy a special place, offering a tantalizing blend of flavor, texture, and psychology that captivates the senses and stirs the soul. From the rich, velvety depths of chocolate to the crisp, buttery layers of pastry, each indulgence offers a moment of pure bliss in a world that often feels overwhelming and chaotic.

So, the next time you find yourself craving a decadent treat, embrace the allure of fats snacks and treats with open arms. For in indulgence lies not only pleasure, but also connection, comfort, and joy. And in a world that can often feel devoid of sweetness, these indulgent temptations offer a welcome respite, a moment of pure delight in an otherwise ordinary day.

Conclusion

The "Macro Cookbook for Beginners" offers a comprehensive guide with over 320 recipes meticulously designed to support and optimize body metabolism. With a focus on macronutrient balance, this cookbook empowers beginners to take control of their health and nutrition journey, providing a wide array of delicious and nourishing meal options. Whether you're looking to enhance athletic performance, manage weight, or simply adopt a healthier lifestyle, this cookbook serves as a valuable resource, equipping you with the knowledge and recipes needed to achieve your wellness goals. Happy cooking and bon appétit.